The Foreskin

and
Why You Should Keep It

By

Samuel M Carnes RT(T) CMD

An In-Depth Look at the Value of the Foreskin, the Benefits of Remaining Intact, and a Debunking of Pro-Circumcision Propaganda

This book is dedicated
to all those who are working to
eradicate the practice of circumcision
from our world and making it fade to a
distant memory. We must keep up the
fight until all boys and men are
left whole and entire as
they should be.

Dear Reader,

In this book, you will hear much information that is going to go against what you may think is common knowledge. I ask that you keep an open mind and read the information carefully. Most other countries in the world do not circumcise and the men and boys there are just fine. Their foreskins are not killing them. Try to overcome what you may have heard or believe. The foreskin is not dirty or gross, nor is it healthier to cut it off. The foreskin is an important part of the body that everyone seems to have forgotten at best or vilifies at worst.

If you read no further or remember nothing else, this is what I want you to take away from this book:

1. The foreskin is an important and valuable part of the body.
2. Circumcision has no health benefits and should never be done.
3. The foreskin is fused to the glans (head) penis and only gradually becomes retractable sometime around puberty. It can happen much earlier and much later. Both are normal.
4. Phimosis is not diagnosable in children under 18 so if a physician tells you your son has phimosis you

know immediately he knows nothing about the intact penis.

5. NEVER, NEVER retract your son to clean his penis. The boy himself is the only one who should ever retract when it feels comfortable for him to do so. When non-retractable, just clean the outside of the penis as you would a finger from base to tip.

6. NEVER, NEVER use soap under the foreskin. Forced retraction and using soap causes many of the problems blamed on the foreskin. At puberty, if the boy is retractable the proper method of hygiene is to retract the foreskin, rinse with water only, and replace the foreskin. Think of it like this – We don't wash under our eyelids do we? Our foreskins are really not that much different in terms of tissue type.

Enjoy the book and happy learning to you!

Table of Contents

Introduction

Chapter 1 - The Basics in Plain Language

Chapter 2 - Proper Care of the Intact Penis

Chapter 3 - Male Circumcision: Medical
Basis or Cultural Bias

Chapter 4 - Medicaid Defunding of
Circumcision: Cost Savings or
Future Expenses

Chapter 5 - Circumcision: An Unnecessary
Procedure that Effects Access to
Care

Chapter 6 - No Reason for Catholics or
Other Christians to Circumcise

Chapter 7 - Where We are Today

Afterward

Introduction

So many people have no idea what the foreskin is, how it works or its benefits. Instead, all they hear are the many myths surrounding it. This book is dedicated to educating about the foreskin and answering your questions about it. Hopefully, this will help to normalize the foreskin and show that not only is it cool to be intact it is also healthier and all around better. First we'll cover the basics in plain language, and then there will be a series of topics relating to circumcision and the intact penis from a series of papers I've written. So let's dive right into the material.

Chapter 1
The Basics in Plain Language

All males have penises. But have you ever studied the penis? For such an important body part it would be beneficial to learn some basic information. Have you ever heard about circumcision? Circumcision is the removal of the foreskin from the penis. Guys who have undergone this procedure are said to be circumcised or cut.

In the United States, for over 100 years this has been a common procedure due to popular custom. It is done for many reasons. These include the false belief that it is healthier, cleaner, more attractive, or because your father is circumcised and that one needs to match. There is also the more vague reason of "it's just what we do in our family." Others have religious reasons. Many Catholics and other Christian denominations erroneously believe it is religiously necessary as well. All of these reasons are false. The rest of the world looks at circumcision with horror, seeing it as the mutilation that it is.

Guys who are not circumcised are intact. This is the proper term to use because these guys are whole and entire. Nothing was removed from them. Terms that you might be more familiar with are uncircumcised or uncut. It is important to use correct terminology, however, to effectively convey ideas. To say uncircumcised or uncut is to imply a state of imperfection as if circumcised is the correct or ideal state. Since this is not the case, it makes no more sense to say a guy is uncircumcised than to say that a woman is unmasectomied. If you are intact, you might have heard terms used towards you such as anteater or elephant trunk. If you are a cut guy, perhaps you have used these terms to tease your buddies who are lucky enough to still have their foreskin.

In the United States, the number of intact guys tends to be much less than cut guys but as people become more aware that this procedure is completely unnecessary, fewer and fewer parents are having it done to their boys. The number of guys born 25-30 years and more ago who got to keep their foreskins is very few but this is only in the United States.

Did you know that worldwide at least 70% of guys are intact? So to all of you intact guys who are reading this: Perhaps you feel like you are the only one, but worldwide you are in the majority.

For you cut guys, many of your parents did not know better. For decades, medical professionals in the United States have been telling parents that they need to have this done. Parents were and still are told the myths that it is healthier, cleaner, prevents diseases and problems and so on. As parents have learned that this isn't true, more and more have chosen to leave their sons intact.

It has been a hard road, though, because everyone wants to do what everyone else is doing and fit in. Many parents don't want their boys to be the only one with a foreskin. They are afraid that if one is intact, they will be teased. We know that boys tease each other, right? If you aren't teased for one thing, you will probably be teased for something else. But I say be proud of it! We have everything we were born with. We were meant to have a foreskin.

What is Retraction?

Retraction is the pulling back of the foreskin exposing the glans (head) of your penis. At birth, the foreskin is fused to the head of the penis and should not be pulled back at all. Over time, it will detach and the boy becomes retractable. Unfortunately, because many people in the United States are so used to the look of a cut penis, they become overly worried about when a boy becomes retractable. Many doctors come up with crazy ages by which they think it should be retractable. They will say one year, three years, five years, etc. Often they will scare parents into thinking there is something wrong if this does not happen.

In fact, the average age is much older, 10-11. Let me stress again, a wide variety of ages is normal. A baby may be retractable. A boy who is 16 or 17 may not be retractable yet. This is all normal. The important thing to remember is if you have a foreskin, no one except for you should ever retract it. Even if a young boy is retractable, there is no need for him or anyone else to clean under the foreskin. Remember, it is not dirty inside the foreskin! When one hits puberty, if the foreskin retracts easily you can retract it and rinse the head and inner foreskin. If it doesn't, then don't worry about it and don't let anyone else try to force the issue. It is completely unnecessary.

Remember this for when you have boys of your own: Never ever retract your son's foreskin for any reason and never let anyone else either. Many doctors will try to tell you it is necessary or that they need to see inside. This is wrong and hopefully as they become more aware of the proper way to handle an intact penis they will stop trying to do this. Retracting before it is completely ready is like pulling off a fingernail. It makes the head of the penis and the inner foreskin like one big raw wound. Protect your boys and don't let anyone do this to them. If you are intact and not yet retractable, don't let anyone force your foreskin back either. Creating this open wound often causes infections and then doctors will say "Ha! You see? We told you that you would get infections if you aren't circumcised!" But no, wrong! They caused it by their mistreatment of the intact penis.

As you now know, the foreskin is not supposed to retract until it is ready and the age is different for every guy. Therefore, you know that anyone who tries to tell you that you or your sons have phimosis or that you should be retracting is wrong. Don't let anyone tell you that you or your son needs to be circumcised. Truly needing to be circumcised for some medical reason is very rare.

Always be on the lookout to prevent physicians from retracting your boys at appointments. They always seem to think they must see under the foreskin. As a retractable intact adult male if a physician retracts to see the glans that is fine but for anyone non-retractable this should never be done. Remember, only the owner of the foreskin should determine when it is comfortable for him to start retracting.

Phimosis is another frequently mentioned argument for circumcision. This is a condition in which the foreskin is narrow or tight at the opening and makes retraction either difficult or impossible. But as you now know, the foreskin is not supposed to retract until it is ready and the age is different for every guy. Phimosis is not truly diagnosable in males less than 18 years of age. Therefore, you know that anyone who tries to tell you that your boys have phimosis is wrong. It is not a problem until adulthood and even then only if it causes pain or discomfort. There are easy ways to take care of it such as creams that can help it to retract, if this happens to be a problem once a guy is fully grown.   Don't let anyone tell you that you or your boys need to be circumcised. Truly needing to be circumcised for some medical reason is very, very, rare and there are other less drastic options. We will talk about phimosis more because it seems to be a favorite with the pro-cutting people.

Cleanliness

Cleaning the intact penis is not hard. Those who were circumcised at birth seem to think that cleaning an intact penis is a very hard thing to do. This is totally false. All that should be done for an intact infant or young boy is to clean the outside of the penis like one would clean a finger, base to tip. The foreskin is not to be retracted for any reason whatsoever. At birth, the foreskin is fused to the glans. This means if one were to try to pull it back to expose the head it would be like ripping a fingernail completely off.

Over time, it will begin to separate and become retractable. This happens at a different pace for each guy. When it is ready to retract the boy himself is the only one who should ever retract it. Even if retractable at a younger age, it should not be retracted and cleaned until after the onset of puberty. Once an intact guy begins washing under his foreskin, it is a very quick and easy process. The foreskin is retracted, and the area is rinsed with water only. Some men use soap, but this is going to cause problems at some point. The glans is sensitive, and soap is going to irritate them. Even if it doesn't right away, it will down the line. Water only is the best way to do it.

The entire process takes no more than ten seconds. Using soap is most likely the primary reason for ongoing irritation that leads to adult males thinking they must undergo circumcision leading to the stories passed around about someone somewhere needed to be circumcised for "medical reasons." Again, it was ignorance and improper care that was the cause, not the foreskin.

Unfortunately, many upon learning that you have an intact penis will say, "Make sure you keep it clean!" This is highly insulting to all of us who are intact and implies that the person speaking thinks that the foreskin must be retracted for cleaning which, as you now know is false. It also indicates that they seem to think you are more dirty if you are intact. Don't pay any attention to such a person because this is incorrect. You continue to rinse under your foreskin with water only (once you are easily retractable), and you will be fine.

Rinsing under the foreskin is such a habit for an intact man to do in the normal course of his shower that making comments like this is insulting and implies that the speaker believes the intact penis to be naturally dirtier.

Chapter 2
Proper Care of the Intact Penis
Introduction

There is a great lack of understanding of the intact penis and its proper care. In the United States, the vast majority of men are circumcised at birth and have been for several generations. Common sense knowledge passed down from father to son has now been lost, since many fathers are circumcised and do not know how to properly instruct their intact sons. Mothers too have lost this knowledge because of the rarity of intact men here in the United States. Even medical personnel are not taught much about the foreskin or how to properly care for the intact male. Many medical textbooks in their illustrations depict a circumcised man and, if the foreskin is mentioned at all, it is usually only in passing and mentioned as something usually removed by circumcision. This has led to a plethora of misinformation that is given out by both the medical community and layperson alike. It is vitally important that we as a society regain this awareness of the functions and importance of the foreskin and its proper care. This lack of knowledge and the improper care of the foreskin are the main causes of problems for the intact male. These problems are easily avoidable if one learns and then follows proper care.

Severe Lack of Medical Knowledge

Pegram, Bloomfield, and Jones (2007) say that "sound knowledge of the anatomy and physiology of the skin is also vital for effective care provision" (p. 356). One could say the same for any aspect of the body. This has proven to be the case nowhere more than with the foreskin. Health professionals learn almost nothing about it other than that it is something usually removed by circumcision. This has led to a great ignorance of the foreskin and its functions and benefits. By further extension, it has led to incorrect and downright harmful advice and practices even by otherwise highly educated medical professionals. Many physicians when any problem arises whether a UTI, bladder infection, irritated glans or foreskin, yeast infection, or anything else, the foreskin is immediately blamed. Circumcision is recommended with no thought to giving antibiotics, rather than leaving it alone, or giving a simple medication. Why should a girl be given an antibiotic for a UTI while circumcision is recommended for a boy? Lack of knowledge and outright bias has also resulted in many erroneous diagnoses such as phimosis. The foreskin is supposed to have a tight opening and not retract in infants, young boys even into the late teen years. This is part of the normal physiological process, rather than phimosis, which cannot truly be diagnosed before adulthood. Alas, since many health professionals do not see many intact males, they do not have the experience or knowledge of how this physiological growth process occurs and instead expect the penis of an infant or young boy to function exactly as that of a grown man.

Previous Work

Kalcev (1964) conducted a study on schoolboy hygiene. Unfortunately, he was not at all aware of the foreskin and its proper care and development. He categorized proper hygiene to mean that the boys were retracting their foreskins. He wanted this to be incorporated into their health education that they all be taught to retract and clean. If they were not retractable, it was something he wanted them to work on and then be followed up with to see if their retractability had improved. He also believed the age where most should be retractable was three and if this was not the case required intervention (pp. 171-173).

Osborn, Metcalf, and Mariani (1981) conducted a survey asking pediatricians what advice they gave to parents of intact boys. They also contacted mothers asking what advice they had been given. Overwhelmingly, both physicians and mothers believed it necessary to retract and that it would retract much earlier than is accurate. No basis was given for the retracting. The paper merely reported the results of the surveys (pp. 365-367).

Another study conducted by Krueger and Osborne (1986) consisted of asking the methods of hygiene and frequency and looking to see the appearance of the glans under the foreskin. They noted adhesions and phimosis but did not specify the age other than to say they were not concerned if the participant was under four years of age. However it is normal to not be retractable well into the teenage years, and it is impossible to diagnose phimosis in a child and young teen. Krueger and Osborne (1986) did not specify who they included in the numbers they considered to have these conditions. In a child or teen who is not retractable, the foreskin is supposed to be adhered to the glans. They also considered any smegma under the foreskin to be an abnormal condition whereas it is a natural process that is constantly occurring in males both circumcised and intact. All three of these things show that they also did not have an accurate view of the intact male anatomy and its normal physiological processes and development.

Since there is a lack of controlled studies on foreskin hygiene, it is, therefore, necessary to build up a proper understanding of the appropriate care based on a combination of understanding foreskin development, the science of skin care, and common sense. It is also important to recognize the cultural biases that exist against the foreskin and not let this effect proper care.

Method of Care

Contrary to popular belief, the intact penis is not difficult to care for or keep clean. In fact, it is the all too frequent overzealous attempts to clean that cause the issues. The best and most accurate advice that all should follow is to leave it alone, never retract an infant or child, and never use soap under the foreskin. Only the boy himself should retract his foreskin when he is naturally ready to do so. No parent or medical professional should ever do so or try to pressure the boy to do so. Before retraction has naturally occurred, clean the outside like a finger, base to tip, and never attempt to retract the foreskin. The intact male, when easily and naturally retractable, often around puberty, can retract, rinse with water and replace the foreskin during his daily shower.

Soap is not necessary and is, in fact, harmful. Retracting the foreskin to rinse is advised only for retractable males who have reached puberty. Even if a boy is retractable before puberty, it is not necessary for him to retract and rinse unless he wishes to. The proper time to begin the practice is up to the individual who is intact. The key point to remember is that it is not dirty under the foreskin. All that parents or healthcare practitioners should say to the intact boy is that "at some point you will be able to retract your foreskin and after that happens, you can retract and rinse with water during your shower when it is comfortable for you to do so." It is important that the intact individual not be coerced or badgered into doing this because the glans and inner foreskin of the newly retractable male are extremely sensitive, and it may be some time before it is comfortable for him. This is completely normal, and there is no harm in the boy delaying rinsing, since the foreskin is designed to help keep dirt out. Forcibly retracting introduces bacteria into an environment that has already been wonderfully designed to protect itself.

Two Main Risks to the Foreskin: Soap and Retraction

Many of the problems that are commonly blamed on the foreskin are actually caused by the incorrect and harmful practices that are encouraged by medical professionals. Because the majority are used to seeing only a circumcised penis, which has the glans exposed at all times, they believe that this is the ideal state. Since the intact penis is covered with the foreskin, they believe this to be less ideal. This leads to the erroneous idea that it is dirty within the foreskin. This is why so many are obsessed with trying to get the foreskin to retract as soon as possible, long before it should. Many parents are told they should be retracting their infants daily and cleaning underneath it. There are several problems with this. First, the foreskin is being ripped apart from the glans over and over again. Bollinger (2007) says that "premature forced foreskin retraction (PFFR) is essentially being skinned alive" (p. 214). This creates an open wound and exposes it to bacteria from which it would normally be protected. This is akin to ripping back a fingernail all the way to the bed in order to wash under it. As one could imagine, this would be very torturous and the parents of any infant who was found with their fingernails ripped back would likely be reported for child abuse, and rightly so. Yet, this is precisely what many doctors tell parents that they need to be doing to their sons' foreskins.

Secondly, the standard of cleaning that has been ingrained in people has been to use soap and water. Soap actually irritates delicate skin and makes it more prone to infection. It also upsets the natural balance that is found under the foreskin and is beneficial. These two main obsessions, retracting and using soap under the foreskin, have caused intact boys and men many issues. A self-fulfilling prophecy is thus created, the penis is sore and irritated, and the parents are told that the best way to prevent this from constantly being an issue is to get their son circumcised. If all concerned would leave the penis alone, these issues would be avoided. The biggest risk to an intact male is the ignorance about the foreskin and its proper care.

Effects of Soap on the Skin

If anything is dirty, we clean it with soap and water. It therefore follows that with the common American cultural belief that the foreskin is dirty, most will believe that extra soap and water is the way to keep it clean. It is sad that when one says to a nurse or other medical professional that one intends for their newborn son to remain intact the first response is often, "Well make sure you keep it clean." This shows the deep-seated belief that the foreskin is inherently dirtier and also implies the notion of keeping it clean by using the norms of cleanliness (i.e. soap and water) under the foreskin. Even if the person who said this does not mean it this way, it is very likely that the person hearing it will take it this way unless they are already well-versed on proper intact care.

Burr and Penzer (2005) say that "the avoidance of soaps for cleansing incontinence dermatitis is fundamental and the use of soap substitutes and emollients is recommended to restore the natural barrier function of the skin" (p. 65). These authors are referring to external skin where the barrier has already been broken down through incontinence. Note that they say avoiding soap is fundamental. Yet, for irritation under the foreskin so many are quick to lather on the soap, exacerbating the problem. Underneath the foreskin is already naturally protected from these situations, highlighting the importance of leaving the foreskin intact and unretracted in the young. The foreskin, when treated properly, provides the perfect protection from this potential skin damage. When the child is older and retractable the appropriate "soap substitute" is water.

Consider that just about every soap, shampoo, or cleanser of any sort usually has a warning on it saying to keep it out of the eyes. We never wash our eyes with soap, nor does anyone suggest that we are dirty because we do not. The skin on the underside of the eyelid and inside the medial and lateral canthus, and around the entire rim of the eye is essentially the same as the inner foreskin area. Would it not make sense to clean them in a similar way? We close our eyes and wash the outside only. So too we should keep the foreskin "closed" and wash the outside only.

Williams et al. (2011) state that "the results from phase 2 of our study confirm the work of previous studies that show that regular exposure to irritants in daily life leads to stratum corneum damage and impairment of the skin barrier" (p. 1311). This study looked at the irritation cause by soaps for hand washing. The fact that soap does irritate the skin on the hands should be a good indicator that soap is going to harm the much more sensitive internal skin of the glans and inner foreskin.

Even with the extra care that is often shown by using gentle cleansers and cloths, irritation of an infant's skin in the diaper area is a fairly common occurrence. This is the external skin! Consider how much more the infant/child's delicate inner skin under the foreskin would be hurt and irritated if one were to try to clean inside there. This is clearly unnecessary, however. In childhood, the foreskin is fused to the glans and the opening of the foreskin overhang (called the acroposthion) is usually quite tight. This end of the foreskin acts as a sphincter, and the repeated outward flushing of sterile urine is part of the protective properties of the prepuce. It allows the urine to leave the body and prevents the entrance of anything from the outside. It has been wonderfully designed to protect the inside of the penis and prevent exposure to the outside world. Dirt and germs cannot get in there unless human intervention harms this natural protection. It is not meant to be retracted at all in these stages of development.

The redness and irritation that results is then often mistaken for an infection rather than a reaction to the soap. This irritation and resulting weakening of the skin barrier make the area more prone to yeast or other infections. Thus, the soap actually causes rather than prevents infections in this area.

Birley et al. (1993), links the use of soaps and excessive cleaning to various skin issues including balanitis. In speaking of non-specific dermatitis (NSD), they state that "a history of fluctuating episodes, with a rapid onset, as well as that of atopy and of zealous washing were predictive of a histological diagnosis of NSD" (p. 402). Citing Fisher (1987), Birley et al. say that "it is possible that the balanitis was due to hypersensitivity to a specific allergen" but they conclude "we could ascribe it to nothing other than frequent soap washing" (p. 402). In concluding the study, they say that "the experience we have gained from this series suggests that an empirical trial of emollient creams combined with advice to reduce frequent washing with soap is an appropriate first line management for patients with recurrent balanitis" (p. 403). Balanitis, a frequently given reason for circumcision, is therefore not caused by the presence of the foreskin but by washing with soap in this area.

A very interesting and relevant point is also brought up by Korting, Hubner,

Greiner, Hamm, and Braun-Falco (1990) when they say that "normal flora growth is optimal at acidic pH levels, whereas pathogenic bacteria, such as S. aureus, thrive at a neutral pH levels" (as cited in Ali and Yosipovitch, 2013, p. 263). If low pH levels are better for normal flora, then by using soaps that raise the pH level we are in fact encouraging the growth of the pathogenic varieties. Ali and Yosipovitch (2013) point out that "candidal intertrigo also preferentially develops in the alkaline environment of the intertriginous areas" (p. 262). An intertriginous area is one where skin is touching skin. Higher pH soaps then, help the growth of infections and these authors point out that there is a "scarcity of low pH soaps, cleansers, and moisturizers available in the US market" (p. 261).

This would explain why those who are washing under the foreskin with soap are more likely to get infections than those who use water or just leave it alone. This increase in the foreign bacteria will likely cause an odor. Using soap, therefore, causes the very thing people think they are preventing by making the environment more favorable to these odor-producing bacteria. This becomes a vicious cycle and because of the odor created many believe that they cannot keep under the foreskin clean. A great point this article makes refers to human behavior:

> Often, patients with intertrigo or acne, believing that their dermatoses are related to poor hygiene, overuse harsh soaps exacerbating the condition and a vicious cycle of further cleansing ensues. Proper education and recommendations on appropriate topicals is crucial in these situations (p. 266).

This is exactly what many people do when confronted with the intact foreskin and if irritation or infection occurs, they blame the foreskin rather than the culprit- the constant cleaning with soap. This explains why when the glans penis or the inner skin of the foreskin become irritated this can often go on for months as the person, and all too frequently, his physician, blames inadequate hygiene and believes that increased washing will solve the problem. When the problem persists, the physician, who has not learned proper hygiene for the intact male, tells the patient that this will continue unless he agrees to undergo a circumcision. Many of the myths that circulate and the stories of ongoing issues leading ultimately to a circumcision are likely this exact scenario. If patients and physicians just knew to stop using soap and rinse with water only these cases would drastically diminish.

Conclusion

Everything discussed can be summarized very briefly. Never retract the foreskin if it is not your own. The boy will begin to retract on his own when he is ready. No parent or health professional should be checking on this nor trying to push the individual to make this happen. It will happen when it is ready, sometime between birth and 18-20 years of age. Phimosis is not a valid diagnosis for a child or teen. Inside the foreskin is not dirty and should never be washed by anyone other than the intact boy/man himself. When this begins is up to the one who is intact when he wants to and then only with water.

Finally, you should tell your sons one time only that in the future he will become retractable and at the time if he so desires he can rinse under his foreskin with water only and mention that soap will irritate it. After telling him this, leave the topic alone. If parents or health professionals keep asking if a boy is retractable yet he may begin to feel that something is wrong rather than that he is completely normal and healthy.

References

Ali, S. M., & Yosipovitch, G. (2013). Skin pH: From basic science to basic skin care. *Acta Dermato-Venereologica, 93*(3), 261-267. doi:10.2340/00015555-1531

Andrews, H. (2012). The fundamentals of skincare. *British Journal of Healthcare Assistants, 6*(6), 285-290. Retrieved from http://eds.b.ebscohost.com.vlib.excelsior.edu/eds/pdfviewer/pdfviewer?vid=8&sid=68eb49c8-a18a-4ac1-88c9-49a08584d8be%40sessionmgr111&hid=104

Birley, H. D., Walker, M. M., Luzzi, G. A., Bell, R., Taylor-Robinson, D., Byrne, M., & Renton, A. M. (1993). Clinical features and management of recurrent balanitis; association with atopy and genital washing. *Genitourinary Medicine, 69*(5), 400-403. Retrieved from http://www.ncbi.nlm.nih.gov/pmc/articles/PMC1195128/pdf/genitmed00029-0074.pdf

Bollinger, D. (2007). The Penis-care information gap: Preventing improper care of intact boys. *Thymos: Journal*

of Boyhood Studies, 1(2), 205-219.
doi:10.3149/thy.0102.205

Burr, S., & Penzer, R. (2005). Promoting
skin health. *Nursing Standard, 19*(36),
57-68. Retrieved from
http://eds.a.ebscohost.com.vlib.excelsi
or.edu/eds/pdfviewer/pdfviewer?vid=
4&sid=ffad2069-2e14-43f2-95dc-
d74d24bb2337%40sessionmgr4003&
hid=4103

Fisher, A. A. (1987). Reactions of the
mucous membrane to contactants.
Clinics in Dermatology, 5(2), 123-
136. doi:10.1016/0738-
081X(87)90014-9

Kalcev B. (1964). Circumcision and
personal hygiene in school boys. *The
Medical Officer. 122*, 171-173.

Körting H. C., Hubner, K., Greiner, K.,
Hamm, G., & Braun-Falco, O. (1990).
Differences in the skin surface pH and
bacterial microflora due to the long-
term application of synthetic
detergent preparations of pH 5.5 and
pH 7.0. Results of a crossover trial in
healthy volunteers. *Acta Dermato-
Venereologica, 70*(5), 429-431.
Retrieved from
http://www.ncbi.nlm.nih.gov/pubmed/
1980979

Krueger H & Osborn L. Effects of hygiene among the uncircumcised. (1986). *The Journal of Family Practice,* *22*(4), 353-355. Retrieved from http://www.ncbi.nlm.nih.gov/pubmed/3958682

Osborn, L. M., Metcalf, T. J., & Mariani, E. M. (1981). Hygienic care in uncircumcised infants. *Pediatrics,* *67*(3), 365-367. Retrieved from http://eds.a.ebscohost.com.vlib.excelsior.edu/eds/pdfviewer/pdfviewer?vid=10&sid=8c0670f9-d836-4143-80c7-312f59480f84%40sessionmgr4001&hid=4203

Pegram, A., Bloomfield, J., & Jones, A. (2007). Clinical skills: Bed bathing and personal hygiene needs of patients. *British Journal of Nursing, 16*(6), 356-358. Retrieved from http://eds.b.ebscohost.com.vlib.excelsior.edu/eds/pdfviewer/pdfviewer?vid=6&sid=68eb49c8-a18a-4ac1-88c9-49a08584d8be%40sessionmgr111&hid=104

Seidenari, S., Francomano, M., & Mantovani, L. (1998). Baseline biophysical parameters in subjects with sensative skin. *Contact*

Dermatitis 38(6), 311–315. doi:10.1111/j.1600-0536.1998.tb05764.x

Wilhelm, K. P., & Maibach, H. I. (1990). Susceptibility to irritant dermatitis induced by sodium lauryl sulphate. *Journal of the American Academy of Dermatology 23*(1): 122–124. doi:10.1016/S0190-9622(08)81204-2

Williams, C., Wilkinson, M., McShane, P., Pennington, D., Fernandez, C., & Pierce, S. (2011). The use of a measure of acute irritation to predict the outcome of repeated usage of hand soap products. *British Journal of Dermatology, 164*(6), 1311-1315. doi:10.1111/j.1365-2133.2011.10246.x

Voegeli, D. (2010). Care or harm: Exploring essential components in skin care regimens. *British Journal of Nursing, 19*(13), 810-814. Retrieved from http://eds.b.ebscohost.com.vlib.excelsior.edu/eds/pdfviewer/pdfviewer?vid=3&sid=68eb49c8-a18a-4ac1-88c9-49a08584d8be%40sessionmgr111&hid=104

Chapter 3
Male Circumcision: Medical Basis or Cultural Bias

Circumcision is a very ancient procedure which gained popularity in the United States only in the past 150 years. Recently, there has been much controversy surrounding the procedure. Most Americans assume that newborn males must be circumcised or else face many problems throughout life. They are unaware that this opinion is not shared by the majority worldwide. The medical community is also divided on the issue. Physicians in the United States tend to recommend the procedure and cite all of the claimed benefits while ignoring their colleagues abroad who disagree. Physicians from outside the United States tend to question the existence of these benefits or at least to question whether they outweigh both the possible complications from the procedure and the benefits an intact foreskin provides. If any issues arise in the foreskin area these doctors tend to recommend treatments that preserve the foreskin rather than remove it as their American counterparts tend to do. American literature is silent about the benefits and functions of the foreskin and so if an issue arises, physicians in the United States often do not to see any value in retaining what they consider to be superfluous. There is a clear bias in favor of circumcision in this country and people claim the health benefits as a reason to justify this cultural bias. There is no need to circumcise. Intact men and boys are just as healthy as their circumcised counterparts and have the additional benefits gained from having a foreskin.

People have many reasons for circumcising their sons including: the father being circumcised, they believe everyone is, they think it looks better, they do not want their son to look or feel different, they want to prevent teasing in the locker room, and they believe it to be healthier. A study found that males born and raised in the United States were the most in favor of circumcision with one comment being, "all I can say is that everybody should be circumcised" and another, "it is healthier for males to get circumcised" (Jia et al., 2009, pp. 94-95). For a small percentage, it is an event of religious significance such as in Judaism or Islam. The most often cited reasons however, are the medical/health benefits of reducing urinary tract infection (UTI), preventing phimosis and balanitis, reducing incidence of penile cancer, reducing incidence of contracting STDs and HIV, and improving penile hygiene.

The American Academy of Pediatrics (2012) writes that "current evidence indicates that the health benefits of newborn male circumcision outweigh the risks and that the procedure's benefits justify access to this procedure for families who choose it" (p. 585). Some believe that lower circumcision rates are bad for the public health, claiming that those who are not circumcised will have a disproportionate level of health problems in the future (Leibowitz, Desmond, and Belin, 2009, p. 144).

One very common health reason given for circumcision is that it reduces urinary tract infections (UTI) which can occur in up to 4% of boys before they are one year old (The Royal Australasian College of Physicians, 2010, p. 10). Schoen (1997) claims that it was once only suggested that UTIs were more common in uncircumcised boys but that it is now definitive (p. 258). He claims that there is a "greater than 10-fold increased risk of UTI in non-circumcised boys compared with their circumcised counterparts in the first year of life" and that "uncircumcised preschool boys and men are also at increased risk for UTI" (p. 258).

Phimosis is another frequently mentioned argument in favor of circumcision. This is a condition in which the foreskin is narrowed at the opening, preventing retraction (Ahmed & Ellsworth, 2012, p. 12). It is claimed that this could be a source of infections, inadequate hygiene, and balanitis (Hunter, 2012, p. 37). According to Schoen (2012), this inflammation of the glans and foreskin occurs in about 4% of uncircumcised boys with circumcision being the best method of prevention saying, "although treatment can be conservative, late circumcision is often necessary for recurrent cases and medical management requires additional physician visits and treatment" (p. 258). Another medical condition is balanitis which is the inflammation of the glans of the penis, the part normally covered by the foreskin in the uncircumcised male, most commonly caused by Candida (Hunter, 2012, p. 36). It is a simple yeast infection.

Penile cancer is a very rare disease, affecting approximately 1 in 100,000 men per year (Frisch et al., 2013, p. 797). Some risk factors given are: being uncircumcised, phimosis, and poor genital hygiene (Ahmed

& Ellsworth, 2012, p. 14). Schoen (2012) states "evidence that circumcision protects against penile cancer is overwhelming" and that "Newborn circumcision virtually eliminates this devastating threat" (p. 258). This seems to be quite a forceful statement for a disease that is so rare. He also claims that the incidence is vastly more common in uncircumcised men (p. 258).

One of the most often stated arguments today is that circumcision prevents, or at least dramatically reduces one's chances of contracting STDs and HIV. It is claimed that "men with an intact foreskin are at increased risk for sexually transmitted diseases (STDs)" and that uncircumcised men have a 3 times greater risk of getting an STD with circumcision reducing this risk by 48.2% (Ahmed & Ellsworth, 2012, pp. 14-15). It is argued that "circumcision can significantly lower the risk of adult males acquiring HIV through heterosexual intercourse" (p. 14). According to the World Health Organization (2007) "Three separate randomized controlled trials in South Africa demonstrated that circumcised men have a 48-60% reduced risk of becoming infected with HIV (p. 22). The researchers even stopped the trials early because they considered it unethical to allow the control group to continue in life without being offered circumcision (Ahmed & Ellsworth, 2012, p. 15). There is also an article which while criticizing the methodology used in drawing conclusions from this series of trials, does not call into question the findings of the studies (Lie & Miller, 2011). Instead, they state that "we do have substantial data from observational research that complement and strengthen the results from the RCTs, [Randomized Controlled Trials] giving us sufficient confidence to recommend circumcisions as a public health intervention to prevent HIV infection" (p. 5).

Another argument in favor of circumcision is that it improves penile hygiene. According to Wilson, Cumella, Parmenter, Stancliffe, and Shuttleworth (2009), "Conditions such as urinary tract infections, cancer of the penis, acquired phimosis, paraphimosis, and candida infection (thrush) can result from poor hygiene" (p. 107). Schoen (2012) says that "US anticircumcision groups claim that genital hygiene can easily be maintained as the foreskin naturally separates, but, in reality, genital hygiene in uncircumcised boys has been shown to be poor" (p. 258). A vast majority of people in the United States believe that unless one retracts and cleans underneath the foreskin daily then it remains dirty and is a haven for bacteria to grow. Since people believe this necessary even in children, they think that is less hygienic for the glans to remain covered by foreskin. Since the foreskin often does not retract until later it makes this cleaning process more involved for those that follow this policy.

There is also the issue of informed consent. Proponents argue that parents can give consent for their children to undergo the procedure. After all, vaccinations are given to infants and young children, who obviously cannot give consent, but whose parents consent for them (Benatar & Benatar, 2003, p. 37). Delaying vaccinations until later in life would leave children exposed to risk of infection and so it "seems entirely reasonable that parents or other guardians of a child's best interests be morally entitled to decide for the child" (p. 37). It is the same with the case of circumcision. Parents are trying to prevent diseases in their children and so for this reason give consent to the procedure in an effort to do what is best for their child.

Now it is necessary to look at the arguments against circumcision. When circumcision started becoming common in this country the fact that many fathers were intact did not prevent widespread circumcision, causing fathers and sons not to match. Children are more likely to notice the difference in size than they will notice presence or lack of foreskin. If they do notice, then one merely needs to explain, age appropriately, so that they can understand the difference.

Many fathers and sons are different in areas other than circumcision status. The father might have a tattoo, different colored hair or eyes, or have a beard. In all of these cases society does not seem to have a problem with this lack of matching so why is it that the penis must match? There is no need to circumcise to match the father. Neither is it a sufficient reason to circumcise to prevent possible teasing. Boys will tease each other over many different things and if not about circumcision status then it will be about something else. Boys should be taught to have confidence in themselves and to be proud of who they are. It is not necessary to cut off a body part just so that they will look like everyone else.

Many people are not well informed about circumcision. Most of the world is not circumcised but many Americans are surprised to learn this. In a study, participants were asked how they felt about circumcision "including the fact that 70% of the males worldwide are not circumcised" (Jia et al., 2009, p. 94). The knowledge level displayed was quite embarrassing with circumcised participants born and raised in the United States shocked to discover that they were in the minority. They also made comments in reference to the number of those uncircumcised worldwide such as "that is a lot of males and a lot of germs" (p. 94). Immigrants were more aware that it is not a world-wide norm and did not feel disadvantaged. Their comments were "I am one of these 70%" and "I am not circumcised and never got any diseases in my life" (pp. 94-95).

Fortunately, the rates are starting to drop in the United States and the societal norm is slowly changing as people become more aware that there is no real reason to circumcise. Rather than follow the majority, it is important that people be educated so that they will see that there is no reason for this societal norm. It is merely a cultural bias. The Royal Dutch Medical Association (2010) calls circumcision "a procedure in need of a justification" (p. 7).

Those who circumcise for religious reason, such as Jews and Moslems, are a very small percentage of the population. Originally, circumcision was much less severe than it is now. Only a small portion of the foreskin was removed. During the second century the religious leaders of the Jewish people became concerned because so many men were trying to hide the fact that they were circumcised. The leaders revised the circumcision rite from being a small snip to removing the entire foreskin, thus eliminating the ability to appear uncircumcised (Gollaher, 2000, pp. 16-17). So even early on, religious circumcisions preserved a large portion of the foreskin.

Physicians from many European countries came together and issued a document refuting four health-related reported benefits of circumcision claimed by the AAP (Frisch et al., 2013). The only possibly relevant argument was that of circumcision preventing urinary tract infections (UTIs) but even this argument "fails to meet the criteria to serve as a preventive measure for UTI" they said (p. 797). They pointed out that "1% of boys will develop a UTI within the first years of life" (p. 797). They also mention that there have been no trials linking a lack of circumcision to UTIs (p. 797). UTIs are rarely serious, and evidence for any protective effect is weak (p. 797).They also show that the risk of complications from circumcision is higher than the chance of getting a UTI. It is extremely telling that the rate of UTIs is similar between the United States and Europe even though the circumcision rate is vastly different (p. 797).

Dr. Rowena Hitchcock (1997) of the Royal College of Surgeons of England says that the paper by Dr. Schoen "reflects the influence of culture and habit on the interpretation of medical practice" (p. 260). She goes on to say that there are alternatives to circumcision that are just as effective for both balanitis and phimosis, yet preserve the foreskin. She indicates that American physicians are much more aggressive and tend to cut off, rather than treat the problem. She believes that this preference for circumcision is a cultural bias rather than sound medical practice (p. 260). She concludes:

> In countries where neonatal circumcision is rarely practiced, and appropriate non-aggressive management of the normal foreskin, with non-forcible retraction and regular cleaning after spontaneous

relaxation of the physiological phimosis, there is no population demand for neonatal circumcision. This supports the conclusion that neonatal circumcision is a social ritual with a grain of medical origin (p. 260).

She also brings up a very interesting point by noting that the incidence of penile cancer is comparable for the United States and Finland even though the rate of circumcision in Finland is less than 1% (p. 260).

Another author notes that the incidence of penile cancer is actually slightly higher in the United States where most men are circumcised than in Denmark were most are not (Benetar & Benetar, 2003, p. 38). This calls into question the idea that being circumcised reduces one's risk of this disease. As for the STDs and HIV argument, it has been noted that while the United States widely practices circumcision, they also have a high incidence of both STDs and HIV.

That the relationship between circumcision and transmission of HIV is at the very least unclear is illustrated by the fact that the US [United States] combines a high prevalence of STDs and HIV infections with a high percentage of routine circumcisions. The Dutch situation is precisely the reverse: a low prevalence of HIV/AIDS combined with a relatively low number of circumcisions. As such, behavioural factors appear to play a far more important role than whether or not one has a foreskin (Royal Dutch Medical Association, 2010, pp. 7-8).

If circumcision is really supposed to greatly reduce these diseases, then the United States with its high circumcision rates should have much lower rates of STDs and HIV than the rest of the world. This has not proven true, however. Is it not much more likely that promiscuity is the culprit? If having a foreskin was really the problem it seems that those countries where circumcision is much less common would have a corresponding increase in incidence of these diseases. The fact that this is not the case is a serious flaw in this argument.

Hygiene of the intact penis is not difficult. Those who were circumcised at birth seem to labor under the delusion that adequate cleaning of an intact penis is a very labor-intensive procedure. This is totally false. In an article on the proper care of intact boys, Bollinger (2007) shows that many physicians and medical websites give either no information on proper intact care or varying degrees of erroneous information (pp. 208-211). For an intact infant or young boy all that should be done is to clean the outside of the penis like one would clean a finger, base to tip.

The foreskin is not to be retracted for any reason whatsoever. Bollinger (2007) notes that "Premature forced foreskin retraction (PFFR) is essentially being skinned alive" (p. 214). At some point in the life of an intact boy the foreskin, which is initially fused to the glans, will begin to separate and become retractable. When it is ready to retract the boy himself is the only one who should ever retract it. Even if retractable at a younger age, it is not necessary to retract and clean until after the onset of puberty. Once an intact male begins washing under his foreskin it is a very quick and easy process. The foreskin is retracted and the area is rinsed. Some men prefer soap while others rinse with water only. Soap is not good for the sensitive skin in this area and will often cause irritation. The entire process takes no more than ten seconds. Unfortunately, many upon learning that one is intact or that one's child is intact immediately say "Make sure you keep it clean!" This is highly insulting to all of us who are intact and implies that the person speaking believes that the foreskin must be retracted for cleaning which, as previously stated, must never be done to a child or infant. To say this to an adult conveys the impression that the speaker believes that he is naturally less hygienic. Washing under the foreskin is such a habit for an intact man to do in the normal course of his shower that making comments like this is like telling him not to forget to wash his left leg or to keep his right arm clean.

Another powerful argument against the circumcision of infants and children is that they cannot give consent for the procedure. In a circumcision, a helpless young boy is strapped down and a very sensitive part of his penis is chopped off. It is gone forever and he can never get it back. An important part of his body was taken from him without his permission. In an article the author correctly notes that those opposed to the procedure "regard circumcision of children to be a form of assault—which is what surgery amounts to when appropriate consent or exceptional circumstances (such as necessity) are absent" (Benatar & Benatar, 2003, pp. 36-

37). These authors make a critical mistake however, by saying, "nor can it be argued that nothing is lost by delaying a choice about circumcision of one's child until he can make it himself" (p. 37). On the contrary, The Royal Australasian College of Physicians (2010) indicates that the supposed health benefits being sought through circumcision "could largely be obtained by deferring circumcision to a much later age (p. 14). Deferring circumcision until one can give informed consent to the procedure is the only ethical choice. It is the one undergoing the procedure who is having an important body part, the foreskin, permanently removed and not his parents. It would be necessary to defer the procedure until the boy reaches his majority to ensure that he is not signing the consent form under coercion from his parents or from a sense of obedience to them.

How can parents take away this choice from their sons? Or even worse, when they are too young to resist, remove their foreskin from them? This is an irrevocable decision. If left intact, they can choose to undergo the procedure as an adult if they wish, but if circumcised, they have no choice, regardless of their wishes in the matter.

Much of the American literature ignores the benefits the foreskin, instead seeing it as a troublesome extra flap of skin. They remain ignorant of what the foreskin provides. The Royal Australasian College (2010) of Physicians states that "the foreskin has two main functions. Firstly it exists to protect the glans penis. Secondly the foreskin is a primary sensory part of the penis, containing some of the most sensitive areas of the penis" (p. 7). The foreskin is not a useless flap of skin. There are many nerves: "The male prepuce has somatosensory innervation by the dorsal nerve of the penis and branches of the perineal nerve" (Cold & Taylor, 1999, p. 17). "Nerve supply accounts for approximately 36% of the total penile allotment of nerve endings" (Hunter, 2012, p. 36).

I can attest to these arguments personally since I am intact. It is lucky that I did not have many physicals as a young boy and teenager since I was unretractable until I was nearly 15 and many physicians in the United States would have diagnosed me with phimosis and recommended circumcision, despite the fact that I never had any issues or problems with my foreskin. They would not have recognized this as a regular physiologic process but would rather have considered it a pathologic condition. Such is the extent of the bias against the foreskin in this country. I cannot imagine having been deprived of my foreskin at birth and I would never choose to be amputated in that way nor would I choose it for anyone else.

Intact men and boys are healthy. They have no more issues with their penises than their circumcised counterparts, despite the hype. The foreskin does not cause more problems than any other part of the body. If there is an issue, it needs to be treated rather than cut off. The foreskin is not a breeding ground for disease; rather it is an important part of the male anatomy that is vastly underappreciated in this country. In the practice of medicine the instinct should always be to treat and to heal rather than to remove. Remember the ancient medical axiom "first, do no harm." The foreskin is causing no problems and is supposed to be there. Therefore it is harmful to remove it for no cause. In the future it will become increasingly clear to Americans that this need for circumcision is a cultural bias. They will eventually come to see that the rest of the world is correct in saying that there is no need to circumcise.

References

Ahmed, A. & Ellsworth, P. (2012). To circ or not: A reappraisal. *Urologic Nursing, 32*(1), 10-19. Retrieved from http://www.suna.org/resources/urologic-nursing-journal/

American Academy of Pediatrics Task Force on Circumcision. (2012). Circumcision policy statement. *Pediatrics, 130*(3), 585-586. Retrieved from http://pediatrics.aappublications.org/content/pediatrics/early/2012/08/22/peds.2012-1989.full.pdf

Benatar, M., & Benatar, D. (2003). Between prophylaxis and child abuse: The ethics of neonatal male circumcision. *American Journal of Bioethics, 3*(2), 35-48. Retrieved from http://eds.a.ebscohost.com.vlib.excelsior.edu/eds/pdfviewer/pdfviewer?sid=6eb4486b-4481-44e8-a9a1-af3b5bfee703%40sessionmgr4001&vid=7&hid=4211

Bollinger, D. (2007). The penis-care information gap: Preventing improper care of intact boys. *Thymos: Journal of Boyhood Studies, 1*(2), 205-219. doi:10.3149/thy.0102.205

Cold, C. & Taylor, J. (1999). The prepuce. *BJU International, 83*(Suppl 1), 34-44. Retrieved from http://artemide.bioeng.washington.edu/InformationIsPower/cold-taylor-prepuce_bju_1999_83_34-44.pdf

Frisch, M., Aigrain, Y., Barauskas, V., Bjarnason, R., Czauderna, P., de Gier, R. E., & ... Kupferschmid, C. (2013). Cultural bias in the AAP's 2012 technical report and policy statement on male circumcision. *Pediatrics, 131*(4), 796-800. doi:10.1542/peds.2012-2896

Gollaher, D. (2000). *Circumcision: A history of the world's most controversial surgery*. NewYork: Basic Books.

Hitchcock, R. (1997). Commentary. *Archives of Disease in Childhood, 77*(3), 260. Retrieved from http://adc.bmj.com/content/77/3/258.full.pdf+html?sid=fea85d25-4c25-46f1-98d9-27cbd4d58baf

Hunter, D. (2012). Conditions affecting the foreskin. *Nursing Standard, 26*(37), 35-39. Retrieved from http://eds.a.ebscohost.com.vlib.excelsior.edu/eds/pdfviewer/pdfviewer?vid=12&sid=6eb4486b-4481-44e8-a9a1-

af3b5bfee703%40sessionmgr4001&hi
d=4211

Jia, L., Hawley, S., Paschal, A., Fredrickson,
D., St. Romain, T., & Cherven, P.
(2009). Immigrants vs. non-
immigrants: Attitudes toward and
practices of non-therapeutic male
circumcision in the United States of
America. *Journal of Cultural
Diversity*, *16*(3), 92-98. Retrieved
from
http://eds.a.ebscohost.com.vlib.excelsi
or.edu/eds/pdfviewer/pdfviewer?vid=
14&sid=6eb4486b-4481-44e8-a9a1-
af3b5bfee703%40sessionmgr4001&hi
d=4211

Leibowitz, A., Desmond, K., & Belin, T.
(2009). Determinants and policy
implications of male circumcision in
the United States. *American Journal
of Public Health*, *99*(1), 138-145.
doi:10.2105/AJPH.2008.134403

Lie, R. K., & Miller, F. G. (2011). What
counts as reliable evidence for public
health policy: The case of
circumcision for preventing HIV
infection. *BMC Medical Research
Methodology*, *11*(1), 1-7.
doi:10.1186/1471-2288-11-34

Schoen, E. J. (1997). Benefits of newborn circumcision: Is Europe ignoring medical evidence?. *Archives of Disease in Childhood, 77*(3), 258-260. doi:10.1136/adc.77.3.258

The Royal Australasian College of Physicians. (2010). Circumcision of Infant Males. *Paediatrics & Child Health Division*. Retrieved from http://www.ccyp.vic.gov.au/childsafet ycommissioner/downloads/male_circ umcision.pdf

The Royal Dutch Medical Association. (2010). *Non-therapeutic circumcision of male minors*. 1-20. Retrieved from http://www.knmg.nl/Publicaties/KNM Gpublicatie/77942/Nontherapeutic-circumcision-of-male-minors-2010.htm

Wilson, N., Cumella, S., Parmenter, T., Stancliffe, R., & Shuttleworth, R. (2009). Penile hygiene: Puberty, paraphimosis and personal care for men and boys with an intellectual disability. *Journal of Intellectual Disability Research, 53*(2), 106-114. Retrieved from http://www.academia.edu/1018031/Pe nile_Hygiene_Puberty_Paraphimosis_ and_Personal_Care_for_Men_and_Bo ys_with_an_Intellectual_Disability

World Health Organization. (2007). *Male circumcision: Global trends and determinants of prevalence, safety, and acceptability.* 1-35. Retrieved from http://apps.who.int/iris/bitstream/1066 5/43749/1/9789241596169_eng.pdf

Chapter 4
Medicaid Defunding of Circumcision: Cost Savings or Future Expenses
Introduction

Healthcare spending is something many Americans worry about every day. As a country, our spending far exceeds that of every other nation. Reid (2010) says that "the one area where the United States unquestionably leads the world is in spending" (p. 9). That being said, everyone worries about trying to save money in this area, from the federal government, to state governments, to individuals. Obviously, it is such an important issue that it is hotly debated in political campaigns as well as among ordinary people on the street. Everyone wants to fix it, or at least to improve it, but no one can agree on exactly how to do this. One hears constant talk about government programs such as Social Security, Medicare, Medicaid, or Veterans Affairs either going bankrupt or, at least, being way over budget. The policies surrounding the creation and governance of Medicare, for example, partly caused the accelerated costs of healthcare in the United States (Morone & Ehlke, 2010, p. 130).

In an effort to cut spending, various cost saving measures have been employed. One such measure has been to defund circumcision and so, in some states, it is no longer covered by Medicaid. According to Andrews, Lazenby, Unal, and Simpson (2012), 18 States have done so thus far (p. 1). This has created much controversy. Some laud this as a good thing, believing the surgery to be cosmetic and completely unnecessary, and as Reid (2010) says, "The last thing we need is a legislative mandate to pay for treatment that is useless" (p. 155). Others, believing circumcision to be prophylactic and of great medical benefit, believe that discontinuing coverage will cause a surge in the infections and medical problems it is said to prevent as circumcision rates decline (Kacker, Frick, Gaydos, and Tobian, 2012, pp. 1-2).

Who is right? Obviously, saving money is a good thing, but it would be bad policy to stop coverage to save a little money now at the price of escalating costs in the future. To get an idea of what is at stake, it is necessary to look at the issues surrounding circumcision. Does circumcision prevent disease? Do boys and men who are uncircumcised have more medical problems and have higher future medical costs or is this all a myth? To compare, it is necessary to look both at the United States population, which is largely circumcised, and the European population, which is largely uncircumcised. By comparing these two populations, it can be better ascertained whether or not these fears are justified.

The Circumcision Controversy

Circumcision is a very ancient procedure that gained popularity in the United States only in the past 150 years. Many Americans assume that newborn males must be circumcised or else face many problems throughout life. They are unaware that this opinion is not shared by the majority worldwide. The medical community also is divided on the issue. Physicians in the United States tend to recommend the procedure and cite all of the claimed benefits while ignoring their colleagues abroad who disagree. Physicians from outside the United States tend to question the existence of these benefits, or at least, to question whether they outweigh both the possible complications from the procedure and the benefits an intact foreskin provides.

Many people are not well informed about circumcision. Most of the world is not circumcised, but many Americans are surprised to learn this. In a study, participants were asked how they felt about circumcision "including the fact that 70% of the males worldwide are not circumcised" (Jia et al., 2009, p. 94). The knowledge level displayed was quite embarrassing with circumcised participants born and raised in the United States shocked to discover that they were in the minority. They also made comments in reference to the number of those uncircumcised worldwide such as "that is a lot of males and a lot of germs" (p. 94).

Due to the statement of the American Academy of Pediatrics (AAP) (1999) which said, "these data are not sufficient to recommend routine neonatal circumcision" (p. 691), it is becoming more common for circumcision to no longer be covered by insurance companies. Opponents argue that this will cost the system more in the long run due to increased health problems of those who are uncircumcised. They believe that lower circumcision rates are bad for the public health, claiming that those who are uncircumcised will have a disproportionately higher level of health problems in the future (Leibowitz, Desmond, & Belin, 2009, p. 144). They will cite the more recent AAP document (2012) which claims that the "current evidence indicates that the health benefits of newborn male circumcision outweigh the risks and that the procedure's benefits justify access to this procedure for families who choose it" (p. 585).

People give many reasons for circumcising their sons but what it boils down to is either cultural, religious, aesthetics, or for the perceived health benefits. A study found that males born and raised in the United States were the most in favor of circumcision with one comment being, "It is healthier for males to get circumcised" (Jia et al., 2009, p. 94-95). This belief in the health benefits has become deeply ingrained in American culture. But is this really the case or is it a myth? Is the healthcare system paying for something that has no benefit after all? Is it really true that circumcision reduces urinary tract infection (UTI), prevents phimosis and balanitis, reduces the incidence of penile cancer, and reduces the incidence of contracting STDs and HIV? To determine this one must look at the statistics and see the incidence of these diseases and issues in both a circumcised and an uncircumcised culture.

Hygiene and Phimosis

One argument in favor of circumcision is that it is said to improve penile hygiene. According to Wilson, Cumella, Parmenter, Stancliffe, & Shuttleworth (2009), "conditions such as urinary tract infections, cancer of the penis, acquired phimosis, paraphimosis, and candida infection (thrush) can result from poor hygiene" (p. 107). A vast majority of people in the United States believe that unless one retracts and cleans underneath the foreskin daily, it remains dirty and a haven for bacteria to grow. They believe that it is less hygienic for the glans to remain covered by the foreskin and will sometimes forcibly retract it before it is physiologically ready to do so, in order to maintain their view of proper hygiene. Since the foreskin often does not retract on its own until later in a boy's development, medical professionals and parents who do this cause damage and often create the very problems they think they are preventing.

Phimosis is a condition in which the foreskin is narrowed at the opening, preventing retraction (Ahmed & Ellsworth, 2012, p. 12). It is claimed that this could be a source of infections, inadequate hygiene, and balanitis (Hunter, 2012, p. 37).

According to Schoen (1997), the resulting inflammation of the glans and foreskin occurs in about 4% of uncircumcised boys with circumcision being the best method of prevention saying, "although treatment can be conservative, late circumcision is often necessary for recurrent cases and medical management requires additional physician visits and treatment" (p. 258).

What these authors fail to mention is that while phimosis may be a pathological condition when the condition persists into adulthood, for infants and young boys, and even into the late teenage years, it is a completely normal physiological process. As a boy develops, the foreskin gradually detaches from the glans penis. This occurs at any time from infancy until young adulthood.

Circumcision and Urinary Tract Infection

One very common health reason given for circumcision is that it reduces urinary tract infections (UTI) which can occur in up to 4% of boys before they are one year old (The Royal Australasian College of Physicians, 2010, p. 10). Schoen (1997) claims, that there is a "greater than 10-fold increased risk of UTI in uncircumcised boys compared with their circumcised counterparts in the first year of life" and that "uncircumcised preschool boys and men are also at increased risk for UTI" (p. 258). According to the Centers for Disease Control and Prevention (CDC), "Overall, UTIs are not common among male infants, with estimates of the annual rate of UTI in uncircumcised infants being 0.70% versus 0.18% for circumcised infants" (Male Circumcision: Other Health Conditions section, para. 5). In opposition to Schoen, Malone (2005) states that studies have only "shown a three to seven times increased risk of UTI in uncircumcised compared with circumcised infants, with the greatest risk in infants under 1 year of age" (p. 773). Singh-Grewal, Macdessi, and Craig (2005) showed that it would take 111 circumcisions to prevent one UTI (p. 853). They also concluded:

> The benefit of circumcision on UTI only outweighs the risk in boys who have had UTI previously and have a predisposition to repeated UTI. As this analysis has used a conservative circumcision complication rate of 2%, if the complication rate were in reality higher the risk–benefit analysis may not favour circumcision even in the higher risk populations (p. 858).

Here they are talking about those boys who

seem prone to recurrent infections. They also admit that they are using a very low estimate, in other words, a best case scenario, when looking at circumcision complication rate. It seems that the number of 111 circumcisions to prevent one UTI is significant. This is 111 surgeries with an estimated 2% complication rate to prevent one UTI that could be cleared up with a simple course of antibiotics. Why treat with surgery when a simpler treatment will work and additionally, will keep a boy or man with all of his body parts intact? Furthermore, girls are more prone to UTIs overall, and they are always treated with antibiotics, not circumcision. Roberts (2011), in the AAP's Clinical Practice Guideline on UTIs, states that "the prevalence of UTI among febrile infant girls is more than twice that among febrile infant boys" (p. 598).

Physicians from many European countries came together and issued a document refuting four health-related reported benefits of circumcision claimed by the AAP (Frisch et al., 2013, pp. 796-800). The only possibly relevant argument was that of circumcision preventing urinary tract infections (UTIs) but even this argument "fails to meet the criteria to serve as a preventive measure for UTI" they said (p. 797). They pointed out that there have been no trials linking a lack of circumcision to UTIs, they are rarely serious, and evidence for any protective effect is weak (p. 797).They also show that the risk of complications from circumcision is higher than the chance of getting a UTI (p. 797). It is extremely telling that the rate of UTIs is similar between the United States and Europe even though the circumcision rates are vastly different (p. 797).

Circumcision and Penile Cancer

Penile cancer is a very rare disease. Some risk factors often given are being uncircumcised, phimosis, and poor genital hygiene (Ahmed & Ellsworth, 2012, p. 14). Schoen (1997) states: "Evidence that circumcision protects against penile cancer is overwhelming" and that "newborn circumcision virtually eliminates this devastating threat" (p. 258). This seems to be quite a forceful statement for a disease that is so rare. He also claims that the incidence is vastly more common in uncircumcised men (p. 258). According to the American Cancer Society (2014), there will be 1,640 new cases of penile cancer in 2014. They report that "Penile cancer is very rare in North America and Europe. Penile cancer occurs in less than 1 man in 100,000 and accounts for less than 1% of cancers in men in the United States" (Penile Cancer section, para.1). According to a report from the National Cancer Intelligence Network (2013), the incidence number for penile cancer in England, Scotland, Wales and Northern Ireland was 1.3-2.0 per 100,000 for the 2008-2010 period (p. 3). The World Health Organization (WHO) (2007) lists the United Kingdom as being 6% overall for their circumcision rate (p. 8). With the vast difference in circumcision rate between the United States and the United Kingdom, one would expect a greater difference in penile cancer incidence than 1 versus 2 per 100,000, if circumcision was really a prominent factor.

Dr. Rowena Hitchcock (1997), of the Royal College of Surgeons of England, says that the paper by Dr. Schoen "reflects the influence of culture and habit on the interpretation of medical practice" (p. 260). She believes that this preference for circumcision is a cultural bias rather than sound medical practice (p. 260). She also brings up a very interesting point in noting that the incidence of penile cancer is comparable for the United States and Finland even though the rate of circumcision in Finland is less than 1% (p. 260). Another author notes that the incidence of penile cancer is actually slightly higher in the United States, where most men are circumcised, than in Denmark were most are not (Benetar & Benetar, 2003, p. 38). This calls into question the idea that being circumcised reduces one's risk of this disease.

Circumcision and HIV Prevalence

One of the most often stated arguments today is that circumcision prevents, or at least dramatically reduces, one's chance of contracting STDs and HIV. It is argued that "circumcision can significantly lower the risk of adult males acquiring HIV through heterosexual intercourse" (p. 14). According to WHO (2007), "Three separate randomized controlled trials in South Africa demonstrated that circumcised men have a 48-60% reduced risk of becoming infected with HIV (p. 22). There is also an article which, while criticizing the methodology used in drawing conclusions from this series of trials, does not call into question the findings of the studies (Lie & Miller, 2011, pp. 34-40). Instead, they state that "we do have substantial data from observational research that complement and strengthen the results from the RCTs, [Randomized Controlled Trials] giving us sufficient confidence to recommend circumcisions as a public health intervention to prevent HIV infection" (p. 38).

It is very interesting to look at the statistics for the prevalence of HIV. If circumcision truly reduced the incidence of HIV by 60%, one would expect to see much lower rates in a country with a high circumcision rate. According to Sansom et al. (2010), the overall circumcision rate in the United States for those born between 1940 and 1979 is 79% (p. 2). According to the website avert.org, the prevalence of HIV is between 0.4 and 0.9% ("HIV & AIDS in USA," n. d.). For all of Latin America the prevalence of HIV is 0.4%, while the circumcision rate given by WHO is <20% overall ("HIV & AIDS in Latin America," n.d.; WHO, 2007, pp. 9, 12). The website circinfo.net further specifies the circumcision rates of some of the countries individually such as Mexico, which varies between 10-30%, Brazil at 7%, and Colombia at 7% ("Rate of Circumcision," n.d.). Circumcision rates throughout Europe are low. WHO lists the overall as being <20% and the United Kingdom specifically, as being 6% (pp. 8-9). Circinfo.net lists

Spain as being 2%, Slovenia as 4.5%, Finland at 7%, and Denmark at 1.6% ("Rate of Circumcision," n.d.). In Europe, there was some variance between countries regarding HIV incidence. Eastern Europe had some countries that were higher such as the Ukraine (0.8%) and Estonia (1.3%). Central Europe was all 0.1% or less and Western Europe varied between 0.1% and 0.4% except for Portugal, which had 0.7% ("European HIV & AIDS Statistics," n. d.). Denmark is especially interesting because, while they have a 1.6% circumcision rate, avert.org gives the HIV incidence rate as 0.2% which is equal to Israel's HIV prevalence and less than the United States; both countries with very high circumcision rates ("European HIV & AIDS Statistics," n. d.).

According to the arguments, countries with lower circumcision rates should have higher rates of HIV, and yet they do not. The incidence in the United States is actually higher than the majority of the countries of Europe and Latin America! The Royal Dutch Medical Association (2010) states:

> That the relationship between circumcision and transmission of HIV is at the very least unclear is

illustrated by the fact that the US [United States] combines a high prevalence of STDs and HIV infections with a high percentage of routine circumcisions. The Dutch situation is precisely the reverse: a low prevalence of HIV/AIDS combined with a relatively low number of circumcisions. As such, behavioural factors appear to play a far more important role than whether or not one has a foreskin (pp. 7-8).

If circumcision is really supposed to greatly reduce these diseases, then the United States with its high circumcision rate should have much lower rates of STDs and HIV than the rest of the world. This has not proven true, however. Is it not much more likely that promiscuity or some other unknown reason is the culprit? If having a foreskin was really the problem, it seems that those countries where circumcision is much less common would have a corresponding increase in the incidence of these diseases. The fact that this is not the case is a serious flaw to this argument. It would seem to indicate that these beliefs are a cultural bias rather than sound medical facts. The Royal Dutch Medical Association (2010) calls circumcision "a procedure in need of a justification" (p. 7).

In looking at the various research articles, it is interesting to note that many things are not based on facts. Many arrive at their basic assumptions, such as the 60% reduction in risk of acquiring HIV number, on data derived from circumcision trials conducted in Africa (Sansom et al., 2010, pp. 1-2). The situation in third world places such as Africa versus the United States or Europe is vastly different in terms of access to healthcare and hygiene practices. Even basics such as running water, food, and adequate shelter are not a given for many in these poorer countries. How can we guarantee that these African trials do not have an inherent bias built into them, whether intentionally or not? As an example, would it not be normal for a health care practitioner to practice cleanliness at the time of the procedure and also to instruct the patient in proper post-op care. This would include instruction in basic hygiene that might be taken for granted in more developed countries but is perhaps a novelty in the countries where these trials took place. Once having learned about cleanliness and proper hygiene, the practice could have continued, and this is what created the reduction in HIV rates rather than from the circumcision itself. This, at least, raises reasonable doubt. Many other things seem to be estimated such as the age of acquiring HIV, the cost of treatment in the future, and life expectancy (Sansom et al., 2010, pp. 2-3). Much of the information seemed to come from mathematical models rather than by looking at the statistics of countries with various percentages of circumcision prevalence. The authors even admit, "the potential impact of circumcision is less well-understood in the United States, where the majority of HIV infection among U.S. males occurs through sexual contact with other males, and the prevalence of male circumcision already is high" (Sansom et al., 2010, p. 2). Yet Andrews et al. (2012) claim, "While there are inherent differences between these populations, there is no reason to believe circumcision would have radically different effects in different populations as findings from prospective studies in the US are consistent with the results from the African trials" (p. 6). The statistics do not support these claims. Furthermore, Van Howe (2004) says that while "several studies conducted in Africa have shown HIV to be more common in noncircumcised men; other studies have shown the opposite, whereas most have shown little or no difference" (p. 591). He furthermore says, "The HIV pandemic in Africa demonstrates distinct epidemiological differences from the outbreaks in North America or Europe" (p. 591).

Monetary Savings and Costs

The question here is whether circumcision costs money or saves it. Some people believe it to be a powerful preventative to disease, indicating that it saves money. Nowhere is this being more loudly touted than in the realm of HIV, which is a very serious condition. Treatments are very costly, and a person can live for many years with the condition. In an analysis, Andrews et al. (2012) used data in South Carolina to determine projected increased costs of treating HIV due to decreased rates of circumcision. They claim a "lifetime treatment cost of $377,360 for each additional HIV case projected" (p. 3). Further, they say:

> We estimate an additional 55 projected male cases of HIV and 47 female cases of HIV in this Medicaid birth year cohort. Using the 2009 reported cases of HIV/AIDS in South Carolina, this figure represents a 13% increase in annual incidence if no

future Medicaid cohorts are circumcised. We project the total cost of these cases in 2010 dollars is $38,635,800 discounted to time of infection and $15,540,800 discounted to birth year. These figures account for lifetime treatment costs for the 2009 birth cohort (p. 4).

At the same time, Andrews et al. (2012) state that "the cost to circumcise males in the 2009 Medicaid birth cohort in 2010 dollars at current reported circumcision rates is $4,856,200" (p. 4). This means they are claiming that in the state of South Carolina, it will cost the system an additional $33,779,600 each year in increased medical costs from HIV, as the price of not circumcising.

One might think that spending nearly $5,000,000 to save $34,000,000 sounds like a good deal. Van Howe (2004) however, using several types of analyses states that:

In every scenario, it was more costly to circumcise. Using the baseline analysis, neonatal circumcision and its sequelae cost $828.42 (3% discount) to $837.59 (5% discount) more than leaving the genitalia intact. Even for the MFS, [most favorable scenario], circumcision was more costly. In all scenarios, the cost of neonatal circumcision is higher than noncircumcision, regardless of the discount rate (pp. 591-592).

He goes on to say that "if neonatal circumcision were cost-free, were immediate complication-free, had no additional days of hospitalization, and had no immediate negative impact on health, neonatal circumcision would still be more costly" (p. 592). Since a greater numbers of UTIs is another common reason given for circumcision he adds, "To make neonatal circumcision cost-neutral, hospitalized urinary tract infections would need to cost $229,564" (p. 592). Obviously, not every UTI results in hospitalization. In fact, most are not serious enough to require that extent of treatment. A UTI is an infection and as such, a simple course of antibiotics will often clear it up quite quickly, just like any other infection. Even in those cases where a hospital stay may be required, it does not necessarily mean that the bill would be that large. Thus, any treatment for UTI that is less than $229,564 results in circumcision not being cost-neutral. Van Howe (2004) concludes:

The analysis is clear: Neonatal circumcision cannot be justified on economic or medical grounds. If the medical community is interested in preserving health and saving money, they should refrain from promoting, encouraging, or presenting neonatal circumcision as a medical option (p. 597).

Conclusion

So what do all of these statistics show? Intact men and boys have no more issues with their penises than their circumcised counterparts, despite the hype. For the most part, the statistics for the various problems associated with keeping one's foreskin are comparable, and in some cases even lower in Europe, despite its much lower circumcision rate, than in the United States. Thus, looking at comparable cultures and levels of prosperity, the evidence indicates that routinely circumcising infant males does not save money. Many of the projected cost increases are mere conjecture using data obtained from faulty trials. Even if the trials had no inherent bias in them, the conditions between the United States and Africa are so different that to apply the statistics observed in Africa directly to situations in the United States would show a lack of understanding of the issues as well be lacking in scientific rigor. It would make more sense to conduct such research in a country with a similar standard of living, particularly in the realm of health care. Just a cursory glance at the European statistics indicates that the foreskin does not cause more problems than any other part of the body when cared for appropriately. It is not a breeding ground for disease, but rather, is an important part of the male anatomy.

The defunding of circumcision is a good cost saving measure. Statistics from cultures largely intact, such as Europe, do not show increased medical problems or costs. This indicates a cultural preference or bias rather than any real prophylactic effect. Instead of using healthcare dollars for unproven treatments, the money would be better spent on essential basic care for more people. The money saved by no longer covering circumcision is a mere drop in the bucket of the savings necessary to get our healthcare system under control, however. To truly decrease costs, many more changes would have to be made. First, we need to look at every treatment, procedure, medication, blood test, and so forth to determine if the practice is truly based on facts backed by evidence, rather than on custom and common practice. Next, we need to put laws in place that prohibit the many frivolous lawsuits that occur. These almost force doctors to order excessive tests and treatments in order to avoid accusations of malpractice and losing in a court of law, rather than being able to use sound judgment as to whether or not a test is truly indicated. Thirdly, we need to simplify the billing system. We have made this so complicated and truly convoluted that rather than being just one of the tasks that we do each day, we have to hire billing specialists. Even these specialists often disagree amongst themselves as to the meaning of various billing rules. Finally, we need to help provide adequate health care for our own citizens before spending money providing foreign aid. While it is laudable to want to help those in far away places, there is an old saying, "Charity begins at home." How can we expect to help others when our own system is a mess, our costs are out of control, and millions of our own citizens do not have adequate health care? By applying these ideas, we may perhaps be in a better position to pursue that elusive dream of a fair and equitable system of health care for all Americans.

References

Ahmed, A. & Ellsworth, P. (2012). To circ or not: A reappraisal. *Urologic Nursing, 32*(1), 10-19. Retrieved from http://www.suna.org/resources/urologic-nursing-journal/

American Academy of Pediatrics. (1999). Circumcision policy statement. *Pediatrics, 130*(3), 686-693. doi: 10.1542/peds.103.3.686

American Academy of Pediatrics. (2012). Circumcision policy statement. *Pediatrics, 130*(3), 585-586. doi:10.1542/peds.2012-1989

American Cancer Society. (2014). *What are the key statistics about penile cancer?* Retrieved from http://www.cancer.org/cancer/penilecancer/detailedguide/penile-cancer-key-statistics

Andrews, A. L., Lazenby, G. B., Unal, E. R., & Simpson, K. N. (2012). The cost of Medicaid savings: The potential detrimental public health impact of neonatal circumcision defunding. *Infectious Diseases in Obstetrics & Gynecology*, 1-7. doi:10.1155/2012/540295

Benatar, M., & Benatar, D. (2003). Between prophylaxis and child abuse: The ethics of neonatal male circumcision. *American Journal of Bioethics*, *3*(2), 35-48. Retrieved from http://muse.jhu.edu/journals/american _journal_of_bioethics/

Centers for Disease Control and Prevention. (n.d.). *Male Circumcision: Other health conditions.* Retrieved from http://www.cdc.gov/hiv/prevention/re search/malecircumcision/otherconditi ons.html

European HIV & AIDS statistics. (n. d.). Retrieved from http://www.avert.org/european-hiv- aids-statistics.htm

Frisch, M., Aigrain, Y., Barauskas, V., Bjarnason, R., Czauderna, P., de Gier, R. E., & ... Boddy, S. (2013). Cultural bias in the AAP's 2012 technical report and policy statement on male circumcision. *Pediatrics*, *131*(4), 796-800. doi:10.1542/peds.2012-2896

Hitchcock, R. (1997). Commentary. *Archives of Diseases in Childhood, 77*(3), 260. Retrieved from http://adc.bmj.com/

HIV & AIDS in Latin America. (n. d.). Retrieved from http://www.avert.org/hiv-aids-latin-america.htm

HIV & AIDS in USA. (n. d.). Retrieved from http://www.avert.org/hiv-aids-usa.htm

Hunter, D. (2012). Conditions affecting the foreskin. *Nursing Standard, 26*(37), 35-39. Retrieved from http://www.nursing-standard-journal.co.uk/

Jia, L., Hawley, S., Paschal, A., Fredrickson, D., St. Romain, T., & Cherven, P. (2009). Immigrants vs. non-immigrants: Attitudes toward and practices of non-therapeutic male circumcision in the United States of America. *Journal of Cultural Diversity, 16*(3), 92-98. Retrieved from http://tuckerpub.com/jcd.htm

Kacker, S., Frick, K. D., Gaydos, C. A., & Tobian, A. A. R. (2012). Costs and effectiveness of neonatal male circumcision. *Archives of Pediatrics & Adolescent Medicine, 166*(10): 910–918. doi: 10.1001/archpediatrics.2012.1440

Leibowitz, A., Desmond, K., & Belin, T. (2009). Determinants and policy implications of male circumcision in the United States. *American Journal of Public Health, 99*(1), 138-145. doi:10.2105/AJPH.2008.134403

Lie, R. K., & Miller, F. G. (2011). What counts as reliable evidence for public health policy: The case of circumcision for preventing HIV infection. *BMC Medical Research Methodology, 11*(1), 34-40. doi:10.1186/1471-2288-11-34

Malone, P. (2005). Circumcision for preventing urinary tract infection in boys: European view. *Archives of Disease in Childhood, 90*(8), 773-774. doi: 10.1136/adc.2004.066779

Morone, J. A., & Ehlke, D. C. (2013). *Health politics and policy* (5th ed.). Stamford, CT: Cengage Learning.

National Cancer Intelligence Network. (2013). *Penile cancer incidence, mortality and survival rates in the United Kingdom.* (2013). 1-6. Retrieved from www.ncin.org.uk/view?rid=1003

Rate of circumcision in adults and newborn.
(n.d.). Retrieved from
http://www.circinfo.net/rates_of_circu
mcision.html

Roberts, K. B. (2011). Urinary tract
infection: Clinical practice guideline
for the diagnosis and management of
the initial UTI in febrile infants and
children 2 to 24 months.
Pediatrics, *128*(3), 595-610.
doi:10.1542/peds.2011-1330

Sansom, S. L., Prabhu, V. S., Hutchinson,
A. B., Qian, A., Hall, H. I., Shrestha,
R. K., ... Taylor, A. W. (2010). Cost-
effectiveness of newborn
circumcision in reducing lifetime HIV
risk among U.S. males. *Plos One*,
5(1), 1-8.
doi:10.1371/journal.pone.0008723

Schoen, E. J. (1997). Benefits of newborn
circumcision: Is Europe ignoring
medical evidence?. *Archives of
Disease in Childhood*, *77*(3), 258-260.
Retrieved from http://adc.bmj.com/

Singh-Grewal, D., Macdessi, J., & Craig, J.
(2005). Circumcision for the
prevention of urinary tract infection in
boys: a systematic review of
randomized trials and observational
studies. *Archives of Disease in*

Childhood, *90*(8), 853-858. doi: 10.1136/adc.2004.049353

The Royal Australasian College of Physicians. (2010). *Circumcision of Infant Males*, 1-28. Sydney: RACP. Retrieved from http://www.racp.edu.au/page/paedpolicy#childrights

The Royal Dutch Medical Association. (2010). *Non-therapeutic circumcision of male minors*. Utrecht: KNMG. Retrieved from http://knmg.artsennet.nl/Publicaties/KNMGpublicatie/

Van Howe, R. S. (2004). A cost-utility analysis of neonatal circumcision. *Medical Decision Making*, *24*(6), 584-601. doi: 10.1177/0272989X04271039

Wilson, N., Cumella, S., Parmenter, T., Stancliffe, R., & Shuttleworth, R. (2009). Penile hygiene: Puberty, paraphimosis and personal care for men and boys with an intellectual disability. *Journal of Intellectual Disability Research*, *53*(Part 2), 106-114. Retrieved from http://www.wiley.com/WileyCDA/WileyTitle/productCd-JIR.html

World Health Organization. (2007). *Male circumcision: Global trends and determinants of prevalence, safety, and acceptability*. Geneva: WHO Press. Retrieved from http://www.who.int/hiv/pub/malecircu mcision/globaltrends/en/

Chapter 5
Circumcision: An Unnecessary Procedure that Effects Access to Care
Introduction

In the American health system there are many procedures that have little to no medical benefit. In some cases, there are better or more effective treatments whereas in others it has been shown that the current practice has no medical benefit but the population as a whole continues to expect it and claim health reasons with no basis in fact. Nowhere is this more true than with the practice of circumcision. There are no medical benefits, certainly none that outweigh the risks associated with any surgical procedure, yet people continue to consider it the norm and many medical personnel encourage it. It is clear that this preference is a cultural bias rather than medical necessity. European physicians and physician groups as a whole condemn the procedure and say that the United States' love for the procedure is not founded on sound medical practice but cultural bias. An example of this is Dr. Rowena Hitchcock (1997) of the Royal College of Surgeons of England who in refuting a pro-circumcision paper by Dr. Schoen says that it "reflects the influence of culture and habit on the interpretation of medical practice" (p. 260). Frisch et al. (2012) issued a document with many European physicians that refutes four health-related reported benefits of circumcision claimed by the AAP and showed how the facts were being misrepresented to support this bias (pp. 796-800).

There is much controversy about Medicaid discontinuing coverage of circumcision in some States. Some complain that they no longer have access due to the cost. This is a procedure that causes multiple problems and does not prevent disease, yet surgery rather than simple care mirrors the American way of favoring extreme medical intervention rather than simply leaving things alone. Simple, appropriate care of the intact penis prevents just about every problem caused by incorrect care and by circumcision itself. Access should be about providing the most effective care rather than whatever people want, regardless of medical efficacy. Doing away with circumcision is in line with the new goal of prevention rather than treating after the fact, since having a normal intact penis prevents more issues than it causes. I propose that circumcision no longer be provided, offered, or encouraged. The money saved and the problems averted will free up time and resources to provide more care to patients who need it rather than devoted to an elective procedure where the patient himself is not even able to give consent. Proper care of the intact male will prevent nearly all of the potential problems people hear about. Circumcision is almost never needed. The stories of persons needing to be circumcised due to medical issues always leave out that fact that it is usually improper care that caused the issues, not the fact of having a foreskin.

Correct Knowledge of Intact Care Promotes Health

Contrary to popular belief, hygiene is not difficult for the intact male nor are foreskins prone to infection. In fact, issues are usually caused by the mistaken belief that it is necessary to retract and wash with soap. Natural retraction often does not occur until around puberty, and until then one should wash only the outside of the penis as one would a finger and never attempt to retract the foreskin. Retracting to rinse is advised only for males who have already naturally become retractable and have reached puberty. It is not necessary to retract and rinse before then even if one is retractable. Soap is harmful and should never be used under the foreskin. It is important to keep in mind that it is not dirty under the foreskin and that forcible retraction introduces bacteria into an environment that is normally internal. It is these very interventions of retracting and using soap inside there that have caused intact boys and men issues, not that they are intact. If the penis happens to become irritated and sore, parents are often told that they are not providing adequate hygiene, and so they begin doing even more intensely exactly what caused the problem in the first place. Soap irritates the delicate glans penis and inner foreskin and causes them to become irritated. This can go on for months as everyone looks for an answer. The physician blames inadequate hygiene and believes that increased washing will solve the problem or often just recommends circumcision immediately. This situation leads to many unnecessary infections, primary care and specialist visits, and ultimately a surgery with all the subsequent follow-up care and possible post-op complications and infections. Leaving it alone is the best solution for a healthier penis. This also helps free up time and resources for patients with actual problems rather than issues that could have so easily been avoided.

Balanitis is one such condition that many associate with being intact but Birley et al. (1993), links the use of soaps and excessive cleaning to various skin issues including balanitis. They say that "the experience we have gained from this series suggests that an empirical trial of emollient creams combined with advice to reduce frequent washing with soap is an appropriate first line management for patients with recurrent balanitis" (p. 403). Korting, Hubner, Greiner, Hamm, and Braun-Falco (1990) point out that "normal flora growth is optimal at acidic pH levels, whereas pathogenic bacteria, such as S. aureus, thrive at a neutral pH levels" (as cited in Ali and Yosipovitch, 2013, p. 263). If low pH levels are better for normal flora, then raising the pH level encourages the growth of pathogenic varieties. Higher pH soaps then, which are most common, invite infection. This would explain why those who wash under their foreskin with soap are more prone to irritation and infection than those who use water or just leave it alone. Odors are also caused by these pathogenic bacteria varieties, and so those who insist on using soap notice more of an odor and so fall into the trap of thinking that they cannot keep their foreskin clean. Medical intervention is not needed. All that is necessary is to stop using soap.

This is why proper education in healthy behaviors is such a crucial part of the process of improving patient health and access. By reducing the need for care for many little things, providers are freed up to not only spend more time with patients that desperately need help, but also to actively participate in educating their patients.

Ethical Considerations

Regardless of the cost savings or spending, the undeniable fact remains that it is a procedure being performed on a child who cannot give consent for a part of himself to be permanently removed. Even if there was a factual basis to all of the talk about HIV and STD prevention, which has not been satisfactorily proven, this still does not warrant putting an infant or small child through the procedure. Only the one whose foreskin is being removed should be able to consent to the procedure. Though it is unethical for parents to choose this based on personal preference and for physicians to push it, this is what often happens. I have spoken to many people who while in the hospital giving birth to a son are asked 5, 10, 15 times when the circumcision is going to occur even though they have been told each time that it won't be happening. This is the solicitation of an unnecessary procedure and harassment. There are those who claim that if one waits until the boy is old enough to make his own decision he will never choose to undergo it. That should tell us something. This is only happening with such frequency because it is being forced upon those who cannot prevent it. Van Howe (2008) says:

> Because circumcision has no medical indication in the newborn period, it is not the first line preventive option for any illness, few boys choose to be circumcised if given the choice and full disclosure is a rarity, and parental proxy consent for newborn circumcision is not valid. There is no reason that circumcision cannot wait until the child is old enough to choose for himself (p. 4).

It is a huge ethics violation to remove a healthy body part based on the fact that it might become diseased, especially, as in the case of HIV and STDs. This would not happen until the child is old enough to give consent. One cannot sacrifice the right of anyone to have a whole body based on a possible illness in himself or anyone else in the future. The very fact that few intact guys would choose to undergo the procedure on their own shows that it is something not desirable to one who knows better. Many of those who do undergo it, do so not so much from a personal desire but because their doctors have worked hard to convince them that it is better, healthier, will prevent future problems, or from societal pressures.

Just in 2014, the Centers for Disease Control and Prevention (CDC) put out a new document where they say that all physicians should counsel their teen and adult uncircumcised patients of the benefits of the procedure (pp. 1-8). I myself have experienced this where physicians try to convince you that it would be better to be circumcised or have at least told me, "I have to at least tell you the benefits." This practice is contrary to medical evidence and completely ignores what the medical community outside the United States says about the procedure. Physicians in other countries have openly accused American physicians of cultural bias rather than sound medical judgment where this is concerned, but American health care practitioners, by and large, ignore everything from outside the country and continue to push the practice on their patients (Frisch et al., 2013, pp. 798-799).

Promotion of Healthy Practices rather than Unnecessary Procedures Increases Access

Devoting resources to helping people and focusing on health and prevention rather than unnecessary treatments helps improve access for everyone. Time and resources should be focused on teaching people more about healthy eating and natural home remedies that have been shown to help. People who are more confident in their health decisions can decide for themselves when it is necessary to come in to be seen by a provider. Those who have been educated know that if they have been around the sick or if they start to get a cold that is beneficial to increase their Vitamin C intake. Often those who have not been taught basic health are unaware of simple things that they can do at home like this. Such awareness would help prevent many unnecessary visits to the doctor's office or emergency room for cases where the only solution is to drink plenty of fluids or let it run its course. If efforts and resources could be spent in educating people, especially parents, in how to deal properly with these things, time and resources in the healthcare facility spent telling people that there is nothing to be done and that it will go away on its own could be drastically reduced. There are many who take their children in every time they get a runny nose but do not seem to be aware that they can stay at home and care for them, thus saving the physicians' time for problems that they can treat, and also help to prevent the further spread of these germs to others, which then prevent others from getting sick, coming in and replicating the process over and over again.

Do Facts Justify Circumcision as Preventative Care for HIV

In recent years, circumcision has been widely touted in popular magazines, newspapers, and on the web as an HIV preventative. The number that has been widely disseminated is a 60% reduction in incidence. This is easily refuted, however, when one looks at the evidence. The three African trials that are always quoted are fraught with bias. According to Van Howe (2008), these trials are not at all reliable:

> These trials suffer from various forms of bias (selection, lead time, expectation for participants and researchers, attrition, intervention and length), improper randomization

and early termination, which amplify the lead time bias. Each form of bias contributed to overestimating the treatment effect (p. 4).

Even those who are proponents of circumcision have criticized the methodology (Lie & Miller, 2011, pp. 1-7). These trials have not been replicated in any first world country. If there was any validity, they would have conducted such trials and loudly published the results rather than continuing to quote only these same three trials continuously. Robinson et al. (2012) say that the World Health Organization has even "suggested male circumcision as an important intervention" (p. 456). They also believe the hype of these same three faulty African trials though Robinson et al. (2012) maintain that "solid scientific research is lacking" (p. 456). In fact, the statistics seem to indicate the contrary. First world countries that are largely not circumcised actually have equal or lower incidences of HIV. The Kaiser Foundation as cited in Robinson et al. (2012) says that "the prevalence rate of adults living with HIV/AIDS in 2007 was 0.4% for Canada and 0.6% for the United States" (p. 457). If circumcision was truly effective in reducing HIV incidence, then countries with low circumcision rates would be expected to have much higher rates of HIV, but this is not the case. Promiscuity is a much more prevalent problem with the spread of HIV than the fact of having a foreskin or not. Activities promoting the reduction in the number of partners would be much more effective in reducing the spread of HIV rather than a mass campaign to circumcise Africa. Even if any of these claims had merit, there is no reason to do it routinely on infants.

Thus, the evidence shows that circumcision does not reduce HIV and therefore, does not help save costs by future prevention, nor does it help free up resources to improve access for others. Once again proper education is going to be more effective. As a comparison, other countries that have universal healthcare do not provide circumcisions routinely, and this has not increased their costs or their incidences of HIV and various other STDs. Why should it be any different within the United States? Van Howe (2008) ends by saying that "as a public health measure the newborn circumcision experiment has already been performed in the United States, and it has failed to protect against HIV infection, sexually transmitted infections, penile cancer or cervical cancer" (p. 5).

Many have tried to say that circumcision is a cost saving procedure by preventing later problems. However, an article by Van Howe (2004) shows this to be completely false. In fact, he says that "if neonatal circumcision was cost-free, pain-free, and had no immediate complications, it was still more costly than not circumcising" (p. 584). He goes on to say that "neonatal circumcision is not good health policy, and support for it as a medical procedure cannot be justified financially or medically" (p. 584). In an effort to improve access for all, it is important that we provide the most effective treatments in an effort not to overwhelm the system with outdated treatments that are not based on sound medical evidence. He points out that "in an era of limited health care funding, close scrutiny of the cost-effectiveness of medical practices has become increasingly important" (p. 584). To help increase access we need to look at each procedure and practice to see what works with the best results. The Royal Dutch Medical Association (2010) calls circumcision "a procedure in need of a justification" (p. 7). This is not the sort of procedure that that should still be offered in a system that needs to focus on effective and efficient care. It is rather the sort of thing that contributes to limited resources, leading potentially to other patients with true diagnosable problems not getting in for an appointment in a timely fashion.

Van Howe (2004) points out that there have been studies that show an increased risk of sexually transmitted diseases (STD) for circumcised males and that they can also get penile cancer (p. 584). Despite the hype that circumcision decreases the risks, the facts do not bear this out. Another thing that is frequently mentioned is that circumcision reduces urinary tract infections (UTI). Circumcised boys get them also, but a Canadian study showed that circumcised boys were more likely to be treated as outpatients (as cited in Van Howe, 2004, p. 588). There is no reason that an intact boy cannot be treated in the same way as a circumcised boy. To give more intensive unnecessary treatment to an intact boy is not an argument in favor of circumcision, but rather that the medical professionals need to be educated in the best course of treatment for both, which should be identical. If an antibiotic is all that is needed for a circumcised boy, this is all that an intact boy needs as well. Other arguments that suggest circumcision is better because of phimosis, smegma, balanitis, are also easily dismissed as a misunderstanding of proper male anatomical development and improper care. Circumcisions are done incorrectly 1-9.5% of the time and must be fixed (Van Howe, 2004, p. 591). This ties up many resources for yet another surgery.

On the other hand, Andrews, Lazenby, Unal, and Simpson (2012) have based their entire cost projections on the belief that the African trials are accurate. They claim as definitive that these trials "have shown that circumcision provides males with a 60% protection" (p. 1). They further claim that "a reduction in rates of neonatal circumcision in states with defunding may result in an increased incidence of HIV infection" (pp. 1-2). They go on to say that "they hypothesized that that defunding of neonatal circumcision will lead to a substantially increased incidence of HIV infection and that the cost associated with these infections will offset the savings from defunding" (p. 2). They then calculate the cost of treating the additional cases of HIV they believe will occur versus the cost of circumcising. They are assuming a lot here. They have also completely failed to look at the European numbers of incidence. European countries are a more realistic comparison because they have a more similar level of health care and socioeconomics to the United States than many nations in Africa. European countries are predominately intact, and yet their level of HIV incidence is no higher than in the United States, and in some countries it is actually less ("HIV & AIDS in USA," n. d.) ("European HIV & AIDS Statistics," n. d.). Over and over throughout their paper Andrews, Lazenby, Unal, and Simpson (2012) mention this 60% protection of HIV transmission (pp. 1-7) but if this was true, European countries should have a much higher rate of infection than they do. Something is wrong with this theory if a country that is predominantly circumcised and one that is predominantly intact both have the same rates of HIV. This seems to indicate that the foreskin is not the determining factor. It is something else.

Conclusion

Sultz and Young (2014) say that "studies indicate that 30%-40% of U.S. health spending is a 'waste' in that it provides services of no discernible value and inefficiently produces valuable services" (p. 295). If this is true, then it is imperative that we take a hard look at what services are actually of value in maintaining the health of the patient. Those that have no actual benefit should be eliminated and no longer offered. If a patient requests something in this category, the provider should take the opportunity to explain that it is of no medical benefit and is therefore no longer offered by the medical community. All medicine should be evidence-based rather than culturally or custom based. If it is not based on evidence we cannot call it science nor is it sound practice. This education provided to the patient is in line with helping to make the patient a partner in their healthcare by helping them to understand what is beneficial and what is a waste of time and resources. This is not to deny patients care but to prevent care that is harmful or unnecessary. In the case of circumcision, there is definite harm caused because a healthy body part is removed with no clear benefit, thus violating a cardinal rule of medicine, "First, do no harm." It is a practice which is culturally rather than medically based. Such practices should not be provided, especially in an overloaded system. This makes access more difficult for patients with real problems. In order to improve access for all, we should only provide care that patients need rather than everything they want. In order to make this acceptable, patients need more education to help them understand the rationale. It will be very important that they understand that they are not being discriminated against but that they are not having their money wasted by ineffective treatments. It will take time and constant reminders until this becomes common knowledge. Staying healthy rather than treating illnesses is the new goal. Doing away with circumcision is in line with this new goal of prevention since having a normal intact penis prevents more issues than it causes and preventing issues before they even happen improves access for all.

References

Ali, S. M., & Yosipovitch, G. (2013). Skin pH: From basic science to basic skin care. *Acta Dermato-Venereologica, 93*(3), 261-267. doi:10.2340/00015555-1531

Andrews, A. L., Lazenby, G. B., Unal, E. R., & Simpson, K. N. (2012). The cost of Medicaid savings: The potential detrimental public health impact of neonatal circumcision defunding. *Infectious Diseases in Obstetrics & Gynecology*, 1-7. doi:10.1155/2012/540295

Birley, H. D., Walker, M. M., Luzzi, G. A., Bell, R., Taylor-Robinson, D., Byrne, M., & Renton, A. M. (1993). Clinical features and management of recurrent balanitis; association with atopy and genital washing. *Genitourinary Medicine, 69*(5), 400-403. Retrieved from http://www.ncbi.nlm.nih.gov/pmc/articles/PMC1195128/pdf/genitmed00029-0074.pdf

Centers for Disease Control and Prevention. (2014). *Recommendations for providers counseling male patients and parents regarding male circumcision and the prevention of*

HIV infection, STIs, and other health outcomes. 1-8. Retrieved from http://www.regulations.gov/#!documentDetail;D=CDC-2014-0012-0003

European HIV & AIDS statistics. (n. d.). Retrieved from http://www.avert.org/european-hiv-aids-statistics.htm

Frisch, M., Aigrain, Y., Barauskas, V., Bjarnason, R., Czauderna, P., de Gier, R. E., & ... Kupferschmid, C. (2013). Cultural bias in the AAP's 2012 technical report and policy statement on male circumcision. *Pediatrics, 131*(4), 796-800. doi:10.1542/peds.2012-2896

Hitchcock, R. (1997). Commentary. *Archives of Disease in Childhood, 77*(3), 260. Retrieved from http://adc.bmj.com/content/77/3/258.full.pdf+html?sid=fea85d25-4c25-46f1-98d9-27cbd4d58baf

HIV & AIDS in USA. (n. d.). Retrieved from http://www.avert.org/hiv-aids-usa.htm

Körting H. C., Hubner, K., Greiner, K., Hamm, G., & Braun-Falco, O. (1990). Differences in the skin surface pH and bacterial microflora due to the long-term application of synthetic detergent preparations of pH 5.5 and pH 7.0. Results of a crossover trial in healthy volunteers. *Acta Dermato-Venereologica, 70*(5), 429-431. Retrieved from http://www.ncbi.nlm.nih.gov/pubmed/1980979

Lie, R. K., & Miller, F. G. (2011). What counts as reliable evidence for public health policy: The case of circumcision for preventing HIV infection. *BMC Medical Research Methodology, 11*(1), 1-7. doi:10.1186/1471-2288-11-34

Robinson, J. D., Ortega, G., Carrol, J. A., Townsend, A., Carnegie, D. A., Rice, D., & Bennett, N. J. (2012). Circumcision in the United States: Where are we?. *Journal of the National Medical Association, 104*(9-10), 455-458. Retrieved from http://search.proquest.com.vlib.excelsior.edu/docview/1312677042?accountid=134966

Sultz, H. A., & Young, K. M. (2014). Health care USA: Understanding its organization and delivery. Burlington, MA: Jones & Bartlett Learning.

The Royal Dutch Medical Association.
(2010). *Non-therapeutic circumcision
of male minors*. 1-20. Retrieved from
http://www.knmg.nl/Publicaties/KNM
Gpublicatie/77942/Nontherapeutic-
circumcision-of-male-minors-
2010.htm

Van Howe, R. S. (2004). A cost-utility
analysis of neonatal circumcision.
Medical Decision Making, 24(6), 584-
601. Retrieved from
http://www.ppge.ufrgs.br/giacomo/arq
uivos/eco02072/vanhowe-2004.pdf

Van Howe, R. S. (2008). Newborn
Circumcision: The Controversy
Revisited. *Auanews, 13*(8), 3-5.
Retrieved from
http://eds.a.ebscohost.com.vlib.excelsi
or.edu/eds/pdfviewer/pdfviewer?vid=
4&sid=9baf5397-7311-4f3f-9a49-
0abc294bc75d%40sessionmgr4005&
hid=4105

Chapter 6
No Reason for Catholics or Other Christians to Circumcise

No book on circumcision would be complete without briefly refuting the religious arguments that people give. I will focus on Catholics and other Christian denominations.

The New Testament makes it very clear that circumcision is no longer an act of any religious significance. The Council of Jerusalem as related in the Acts of the Apostles says that circumcision, among other practices, is no longer required. There are many other instances when St Paul makes this quite clear in his Epistles.

For Catholics specifically, it has been the consistent teaching since the time of Christ that circumcision is no longer required and is forbidden. Many church fathers, canonized saints, popes, and councils make reference to it being forbidden throughout the centuries. This has been consistent right up to the present day with the current Catechism of the Catholic Church (1994) states: "Except when performed for strictly therapeutic medical reasons, directly intended amputations, mutilations, and sterilizations performed on innocent persons are against the moral law" (para. 2297). Some will argue that circumcision is therapeutic but as has been shown circumcision is only necessary on extremely rare cases. One cannot make the extreme exception the rule. Routine circumcision without an extremely pressing immediate need, therefore, qualifies this procedure as mutilation and is therefore forbidden.

When one looks at the multitude of statements forbidding circumcision throughout the Church's history one cannot now claim that the Church is excluding circumcision when they condemn mutilation. This is a clear example of the American bias coloring their view. It is absolutely unacceptable to hear Catholics and other Christians say that they did it for "religious reasons." You have no religious reason to do so.

Even more recently Pope Benedict XVI (2007) said:

> Together with Paul, he then went to the so-called Council of Jerusalem where after a profound examination of the question, the Apostles with the Elders decided to discontinue the practice of circumcision so that it was no longer a feature of the Christian

identity (cf. Acts 15: 1-35). It was only in this way that, in the end, they officially made possible the Church of the Gentiles, a Church without circumcision; we are children of Abraham simply through faith in Christ (para. 9).

It is clear from these facts that neither Catholics nor any other Christian denomination can legitimately accept circumcision as morally acceptable.

References

Benedict XVI. (January, 2007). *General Audience.* Retrieved from http://w2.vatican.va/content/benedict-xvi/en/audiences/2007/documents/hf_ben-xvi_aud_20070131.html

Catholic Church. (1994). *Catechism of the Catholic Church.* Vatican City: Libreria Editrice Vaticana.

Chapter 7
Where We are Today

Today there is still much work to be done. The information about the benefits of the foreskin is getting out there. We are slowly dispelling the myths and showing people that there is no point to circumcision. Those in favor of circumcision are fighting back, trying to vilify the foreskin even more and trying to vilify us and make us look like ignorant fools. We must be doing something right!

In an effort to bolster support for their outdated views they come up with more and more new "medical reasons" to circumcise. They have tried hygiene, penile cancer, HIV, and now I have started hearing that they try to claim that the foreskin affects or leads to prostate cancer. This is laughable because it is so absurd. They are really getting desperate!

Another thing that they are now doing is to try and encourage intact teens and adults of the supposed benefits. It's almost as if they think that since they lost their chance to get their way and circumcise everyone at birth they are now going to try and persuade intact males that they have a problem or a potential problem. They act as if the foreskin is a bomb just waiting to explode with disease. They have no valid reason for this. It is just another example of them using the same old myths and misinformation campaign to push the practice. Unfortunately, many might believe it, thinking the physician knows best and cave to the pressure. They might even have a little irritation from using soap and the doctor tells them that circumcision is the answer. Voila! Now we have another story to spread around of how this random person "had to be circumcised for medical reasons." I myself have had physicians say that they need to at least tell me the benefits of getting circumcised. But you know what? There aren't any so give it up already! We are gaining ground, and the truth is getting out there. Keep up the fight.

There is absolutely no reason to be circumcised! STAY INTACT and be proud of it!

References

Centers for Disease Control and Prevention. (2014). *Recommendations for providers counseling male patients and parents regarding male circumcision and the prevention of HIV infection, STIs, and other health outcomes.* 1-8. Retrieved from http://www.regulations.gov/#!documentDetail;D=CDC-2014-0012-0003

Afterward

Thank you for reading this book. I hope I have convinced you that circumcision is wrong and should never be practiced. I hope I have helped you see through the lies and propaganda used to perpetuate this horrible practice.

I have plans for a second book in which I plan to include more on:

1. Anatomy and Physiology of the foreskin and the intact male
2. The ethics involved and lack of consent of the infant with regards to circumcision
3. More on diseases and the statistics
4. More in-depth discussion and many quotes for Catholics and other Christians on why circumcision is forbidden and definitely not required.

Perhaps there will be some other aspects as well, as I continue to research and write more on this important topic.

Made in the USA
Charleston, SC
18 December 2015